WHEN YOU ARE DEPRESSED

DIFFICULT TIMES SERIES

WHEN YOU ARE DEPRESSED

DAVID ALLEN SORENSEN AND
BARBARA DEGROTE-SORENSEN

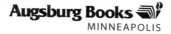
MINNEAPOLIS

*For all the wounded healers
who have emerged from their own depression
and now freely come alongside others
who walk in emotional darkness:
Faith. Courage. Peace.*

Large-quantity purchases or custom editions of this book are available at a discount from the publisher. For more information, contact the sales department at Augsburg Fortress, Publishers, 1-800-328-4648, or write to: Sales Director, Augsburg Fortress, Publishers, P.O. Box 1209, Minneapolis, MN 55440-1209.

Scripture passages are from the New Revised Standard Version and the Revised Standard Version of the Bible, copyright © 1946, 1952, 1971, 1989 by the Division of Christian Education of the National Council of the Churches of Christ in the USA. Used by permission.

Cover design by David Meyer
Book design by Jessica A. Klein

ISBN 0-8066-4420-6

The paper used in this publication meets the minimum requirements of American National Standard for Information Sciences—Permanence of Paper for Printed Library Materials, ANSI Z329.48-1984. ♾™

Manufactured in the U.S.A.

06   05   04   03   02   1   2   3   4   5   6   7   8   9   10

§ *Contents* §

Introduction: What's It All About?   7

Chapter One: How Do I Know if I'm Depressed?   12

Chapter Two: What Causes Depression?   17

Chapter Three: Where Do I Go to Find Help?   21

Chapter Four: What More Can I Do to Help Myself? 27

Chapter Five: Depression—A Family Perspective   38

Chapter Six: How Do I Get Back on Track?   46

A Note to Clergy, Counselors, and Other Caregivers   50
Notes   52
Works Cited   53
Additional Resources   54
Internet Resources   55

§ *Introduction* §
What's It All About?

As you take up this book, what are you longing for? Relief from depression? Assurances that you can endure this present depression? Resources to help you rise above depression? Help for a loved one? We've written this book of spiritual care to help you in any or all of these areas.

Whether you long for healing or the ability to endure, under it all you may well be longing for God.

"As a deer longs for flowing streams, so my soul longs for you, O God. My soul thirsts for God, for the living God. When shall I come and behold the face of God? My tears have been my food day and night . . ." (Psalm 42:1-3).

These words come from the same depressed person who continues with:

"My soul is cast down within me."

"I say to God, my rock, 'Why have you forgotten me?'"

"Why must I walk about mournfully?"

"Why are you cast down, O my soul, and why are you disquieted within me?"

That is how I (David) felt and thought during several challenging times in my life—sadness, deep sadness, even depression. With appropriate help, the smoothing touch of time, and especially the intimate healing of God, I'm much better now, though I suspect some of us go through life, for various reasons, with a persistent low-grade depression even when we're at our healthiest.

I've found that people who have lived with depression can discover a deep bond as they share their lives with each other. In the words of Psalm 42:7, "Deep calls to deep." May something deep within you connect with something deep within us—deep where it hurts, deep where the healing will come, deep where God is.

WHAT THIS BOOK IS

When You Are Depressed is a book of spiritual care for depression that is informative, interactive, and solution-focused. We want to help you deal with your depression and limit its impact on those around you. Those who have emerged from one or two depression episodes may find the book useful for developing new skills and insights.

First, we introduce you briefly to some of the causes and types of depression as well as treatments and other help you can seek out to deal with it. We also describe the unique place of spiritual care as an important part of anyone's overall mental and physical health.

Then we direct you to places where healing can happen, and to some things you can try yourself to help with your sadness or depression. These steps may be enough to deal effectively with a mild to medium depression. Most depressions fall into these categories. If you have a deeper, more difficult depression, consider this process a new beginning leading to further help.

Next, because experiences of depression often happen within a family system of one kind or another, we address the role of family and friends. We also share suggestions and stories from others, including ourselves, who have been there for each other. We answer the question: "Where do I go from here?" We direct you to resources beyond the scope of this small book and send you off with a prayer and a blessing.

WHAT THIS BOOK IS NOT

This is not the place to seek extensive information about diagnosis and treatment of depression. See the Additional Resources section for a description of other more substantive assistance.

This book is not intended to be a substitute for contact with others. We envision it as a starting place that can lead you to other kinds of help and contacts with others, perhaps a pastor or other counselor. If we can encourage you to reach out to others, we believe your time working through *When You Are Depressed* will have given you a good start in understanding and being able to articulate your own situation.

This small book can't do *everything*. But it can and will do *something*. And that *something* may be just what you need to begin moving toward greater health in every way.

Acknowledgments

I (David) would like to thank some of the people who have taught and mentored me in the ways of the inner person:

Margaret Reed and Wayne Sandee, for wisely guiding me into a degree in social work so I could later hit the ground running as a young pastoral counselor.

Hugh Kaste and Lori Ruthenbeck, my supervisors during a life-changing counseling internship at Lutheran Social Service of Minnesota.

Dan Simundson, Warren Quanbeck, Bill Hulme, Lee Griffin, Bill Smith, and "Papa" Smits, doctors of the soul, teachers I sought out when possible at Luther Seminary in St. Paul.

Bill Miller and Wally Peterson, my clinical pastoral education supervisors at Fairview-University Hospital, Riverside Campus of Minneapolis.

Fr. Gus Biehl and Sr. Michaela Hedican, spiritual directors and friends who blessed us with many gifted insights.

The Benedictine monks of St. John's Abbey in Collegeville, Minnesota, for their extravagant hospitality and a place to pray, heal, think deep thoughts, and write.

Andrew Hanson, Blanche Tirk, and the many other gifted servants and ministers I've worked with who have modeled compassionate care, thereby molding my counseling ministry and my life during more than twenty years of ordained service.

Our family of Salem Lutheran Church in St. Cloud, Minnesota, for inviting us to share in an all too rare, Spirit-led freshness and servanthood. Discovering the many outward expressions of our inner life with Christ has never been more fun.

Finally, our heartfelt thanks to Howard Stone, Professor of Pastoral Theology and Pastoral Counseling at Brite Divinity School, Texas Christian University. An authority on ministry to the depressed, and author of several books that were particularly useful for this project (see the Works Cited section), Dr. Stone generously provided time for personal consultations and a critique of our manuscript. Many of the most useful aspects of this book are based on his model for brief pastoral counseling; any errors or oversights are our own.

> "By the tender mercy of our God,
> the dawn from on high will break upon us,
> to give light to those who sit in darkness
> and in the shadow of death,
> to guide our feet into the way of peace."
> (Luke 1:78-79)

§ Chapter One §

How Do I Know if I'm Depressed?

We asked a pastor who counsels many people with depression, "What does depression look like when it walks through your door?" She replied, "It often wears the face of shame. Sometimes I'll hear:

"I'm probably just being a baby, but . . ."

"I'm sorry to waste your time, but . . ."

"I should be able to handle this, but . . ."

It's the part that comes after the "but" that needs the listening. The depressed person knows something is wrong. The real message is often the most difficult to communicate. Sometimes it takes courage to hurdle the fear and invisible social stigma often associated with depression to finally own it, name it, claim it, and move gently forward.

It's easier to talk about what depression isn't rather than what it is. It's not just feeling "stressed-out." It's not just a bad mood, the blues, or symptoms due to PMS. It's not being edgy, nervous, or anxious. It's not just a bad day or experiencing grief over a sudden loss. These are feelings that we all have at times. When you face a serious loss or a series of difficult experiences, a minor depression would be a natural response.

A major depression is longer lasting. It could feel much like a minor depression, but it lasts for two weeks, sometimes much longer. Major depression involves a chemical imbalance in the brain that affects our daily functioning. This imbalance takes once pleasurable activities and robs them of their joy. It delivers a feeling of helplessness and hopelessness. The depressed person tends to sleep and/or eat too much or too little. Personal hygiene often slips. There is often a feeling of extreme anxiety or foreboding. Some may experience physical symptoms, such as chronic aches and pains or digestive problems. Early stages of depression, especially in teenagers, can be shown in irritability or angry words and actions.

Those who have experienced depression talk about a deep, black hole inside themselves from which there appears to be no escape. Depression is not the same as grief. There are no stages. It lingers. It seldom goes away by itself.

The following exercise may help you determine if you or a loved one has an ordinary minor depression or a more serious major episode.

If you are unsure about whether you have depression, answer the following questions yes or no:

1. I feel downhearted and sad almost all the time.
2. I do not enjoy the things that I used to.
3. I have felt so low I've thought about suicide.
4. I feel that I am not useful or needed.
5. I am losing weight.
6. I have trouble sleeping through the night.
7. I am restless and cannot keep still.
8. My mind is not as clear as it used to be.
9. I get tired for no reason.
10. I feel hopeless about the future.

You may be suffering from major depression if you answered yes to the first two questions and if your symptoms have persisted for at least two weeks. If you have been feeling depressed and answered yes to at least two of questions 4 through 10, you may have a mild form of depression. Talk to your doctor. Regardless of how you answered the other questions, if you answered yes to question 3, call your doctor or a suicide hotline (look in the Yellow Pages of the phone book under "Crisis Intervention") immediately for help. (From *Harvard Medical School Family Health Guide* by Anthony Komaroff [Simon & Schuster, 1999], p. 396)

Depression is on the increase in Western Europe, North America, the Middle East, and Asia, affecting all ages, socioeconomic levels, the educated and non-educated, religious and non-religious. It is the number one mental health problem in the United States. About one in five adults will experience a major depression in their lifetime; women are twice as likely to experience depression as men. It is a growing problem among adolescents. Sometimes there is a precipitating transition or event, sometimes not. A major depression seldom goes away by itself. The greatest danger of depression is suicide.

If you think you or someone you care about may have a major depression, this little book is a start, but it is not enough. Seek further help in the form of a counselor or doctor. Do it knowing that you are not alone; though its effects reveal themselves in highly individual ways, depression has been called the common cold of mental health.

On the first day of my counseling internship with Lutheran Social Service of Minnesota, I (David) was led to the file drawers where many of the notes and test results of the most recent clients were kept. "To familiarize you with the range of counseling we do at this agency," my supervisor said, "I'd like you to spend two days just reading about the kinds of personal struggles our people bring to us. This is a rare opportunity we're offering you, but I think it's an important part of your training."

That would have been a memorable experience under any circumstances, but it happened that the counseling agency was housed in the church where I had grown up. I knew many of these people, or at least knew of them. The only thing odd about the group was that there was nothing odd about them. They seemed like a cross-section of everyone in town. I read for two days about their hurts, most of them dealing with a deep sadness or depression in combination with other issues. Though I was surprised at first to find that many people who seemed to have it pulled together were seeking help, I found it oddly comforting. Inner struggles were as common as the lament psalms in the Bible.

I think I was healed that week of some of my need to keep appearances up when life becomes challenging. *What will the neighbors think?* I'm convinced that at any given time, a bunch of your neighbors and mine—call them a *pride* of neighbors—have troubles of their own but hide them with varying degrees of success. That shift in my opinion about people dealing with depression would pay dividends years later. I would come to know what it was like to be on both sides of a counselor's desk.

Barbara picks up the story:

David had been feeling low off and on for several months. Many of the signs of depression were there. Sleep disorder. Persistent sadness. Withdrawing. Short-tempered or unresponsive. Weight change. It wasn't uncommon for me to come home and find him in bed, exhausted from dealing with his life's normal expectations. He had gone through too many significant grieving experiences in just a few months. He was physically and emotionally worn down. Looking back, I'm not sure why I didn't do something sooner.

We talked a lot about the changes in his behavior but shied clear of the word "depression." It didn't seem bad enough to seek outside help yet. If I had had a checklist of warning signs, maybe I would have seen it coming. I thought he could get himself out of it, just a situational thing that would pass as soon as he got a vacation. In the meantime, I just coped and waited and denied all the warning signs.

Eventually, he went through a battery of medical and psychological tests, got directed to the help he needed, and made a good recovery back into a healthy, creative life and ministry. But we wish we had known then what we know now about the causes and symptoms of depression and what we can do about it.

§ Chapter Two §
What Causes Depression?

No one can say clearly why one person becomes depressed and another does not. Today, it is mostly thought that depression is a medical condition tied to an imbalance in the complicated chemicals in our brains that monitor mood. A low serotonin level is one of the chemicals often linked to major depression. How or why certain brain chemicals get depleted is still under study.

There is still much research being done as to the genetic and pre- and post-existing environmental influences that contribute to depression. An imbalance in brain chemistry will affect how we see life and our place in it. Depression can be caused by both past and present life situations or genetic dispositions, or a combination of the two. Sometimes a major depression can be related to a stressful event or a string of events that suppress our body's ability to produce the proper chemicals that communicate to the rest of the body that life is good. Other times, depression appears for no apparent reason at all. Depression may run in families.

In some cases, the depression comes from within, caused by a chemical imbalance, fatigue, stroke, or a variety of physical or internal illnesses. Other types of depression stem from other events, such as stressful situations or emotional conflict.

Such external conflicts may be broken down further, analyzing the depression from either a spiritual or psychological core. Psychological depression affects persons who have learned unhealthy patterns to deal with life's stresses, using sadness to manipulate, for example. Self-esteem issues could also fall under this category. Spiritual depression encompasses issues of guilt and shame, anger toward God, and the need for confession and forgiveness. In most cases of depression, the causes of depression often involve two or three areas: physical, psychological, and/or spiritual.[1]

One of the most recurring themes in the study of external depression is loss. According to Roy Fairchild, "Failure at work and school, rejection, death of a loved one, physical disability, marital conflict, financial difficulty, being severed from a familiar role, are common 'triggers' for depression."[2]

Fairchild goes on to explain that even success can be a loss. When difficult goals have been achieved, people often discover a sudden sadness. It was the striving toward the goal that gave life its impetus, its meaning. When the goal has been reached, the continued striving lacks purpose. Without meaning in our lives, without purpose, we flounder.

Loss of faith or feeling cut off from God often can accompany or trigger depression. The depressed person asks, "Where is God in my suffering?" or "Why wasn't God there for me?" Even Jesus from the cross cried out, "My God, my God, why have you forsaken me?" Such feelings of being abandoned by God leave us shaken and searching for self-worth and meaning. We can barely whisper the big question: If God forsakes us, what then?

Unacknowledged resentment, anger, or guilt toward oneself or another can also trigger depressive tendencies. Anger turned inward is a well-known cause of depression. Unforgiven actions in ourselves and others, dwelt upon over time, can send us spiraling downward.

Such thoughts feed on themselves. We begin to exhibit some of the negative self talk associated with depression. The depressed person may cling to such false beliefs as:

• "I have no power in my situation."
• "No one finds me attractive anymore."
• "I have no friends because I am not lovable."

As a result of such thinking, there may be a hairpin trigger on many emotions and behaviors. Anger may become manipulative, causing others to see our suffering and perhaps feel sorry for us. Such thinking and accompanying behavior often results in others pulling back from us, and the cycle continues. Feeling distracted is common in mild and medium depressions, so do what contributes to health despite your feelings. Persistent negative thoughts can result in negative consequences. Such negative self-talk pushes away the gift of grace from those who need to hear it most. Feeling unfit or unworthy, our bodies respond by depleting the very chemicals that help us acknowledge joy, peace, patience, and a sense of well-being. We become our own worst enemy.

Understanding the causes of depression may be of some help, but probably won't work as a cure-all for most depressed people. At some point, we may not be able to pull ourselves up by our own psychological bootstraps. We may need to run the risk of asking for help.

The good news is that advances in physical and mental health care make depression highly treatable. More than eighty percent of those who experience depression overcome it through medical and/or talk therapy. Those who experience depression today have reason to be hopeful.

§ Chapter Three §
Where Do I Go to Find Help?

If you wonder if you or a loved one may be depressed, most experts suggest a thorough physical examination to see if there is any physical reason for the depression. Getting a good physical may alleviate some of the anxious thinking associated with depression. A doctor can also help to diagnose depression. Early diagnosis, as with other illnesses, can often decrease the length and severity of the problem. Most depressed people respond well to treatment with anti-depressant medicines, talk therapy or, preferably, a combination of the two.

The new generation of anti-depressant medications called SSRIs (Selective Serotonin Re-uptake Inhibitors), introduced in 1988, are as effective or better than previous medications, but are safer and have fewer side effects. They restore the brain's neurotransmitters—including serotonin, norepinephrine, and dopamine—chemical messengers that communicate to a person that life is good. The medication is typically continued for a minimum of several months, with the option of longer-term therapy to be determined with a doctor's advice. When normal brain functioning is restored, life doesn't just seem better, one sleeps better and rises to greet the new day with more happiness, concentration, and energy.

Although it may be difficult, it is important to acknowledge the need for help and ask for it. Seeing depression as a disease with physical symptoms is still being misunderstood by some. As unnecessary as that is, there still remains somewhat of a stigma when it comes to depression.

Missouri Senator Tom Eagleton, George McGovern's 1972 presidential running mate, withdrew his candidacy after it became publicly known that he had once been treated for depression. Some thought he wasn't "strong" enough for the position.

Barbara shares:

One well-intentioned friend told us that a friend of hers had gone through a time of depression, then his company didn't want him back. She didn't stop to think of the impact that story might have on us as we considered David's experience of depression in the midst of doing his job. A neighbor came right out and asked me how a pastor could get depressed. It was a fear-based question. If pastors can become depressed, what about the rest of us? There's still a feeling, when it comes to depression, that we should be able to pull ourselves out of it if we just try harder.

While there are things we can do to help ourselves in our depression (see chapter 4), its very symptoms deny many the strength to try. It is then that we must ask for the help we need. Depression, when understood in the context of brain chemicals and not moral weakness, allows a person to maintain dignity, moving toward health and away from the baggage of shame and guilt leftover from a less enlightened time.

So, where to begin? Once you've had a physical examination and are taking medication and seeing a professional counselor, continue to network and add to your support system. Begin with a few small steps.

REALIZE THAT YOU ARE NOT ALONE IN YOUR DEPRESSION

Many people from the Bible suffered from depressive symptoms. Elijah refused to eat or drink and found himself alone in a cave wishing for death. God first fed him and strengthened him, and later led him to a widow's house. She, too, was suffering under her depressive conditions. Down to her last resources, she planned to prepare a final meal and then prepare for death. She shared her story and bread with Elijah, and they were strengthened by one another's experience and the presence of God. Life continued. It has for many people who have suffered from depression at one time or another.

TALK TO OTHER PEOPLE

For those with a mild depression, simple things like talking to a friend or pastor, exercising, or seeking social contacts are useful. This can take courage. The illness will try to hold you back. This is a time to give yourself grace. Set small doable goals. Each attempt to connect outside your depressed feelings will give you courage to try again. Let others know you need their support.

JOIN A DEPRESSION SUPPORT GROUP

A telephone call to a local counseling center or church should provide you with guidance in tracking down support groups in your area. An effective support group gently invites people out of their isolation, allows them to tell their stories and focus on their healing. A typical support group lasts from sixty to ninety minutes. It is an open group where health and healing can come.

"They told me I didn't have to say anything," one person stated upon visiting her church's support group for the first time. For some, just listening to other people's stories with nothing expected from them in return provides a safe place to look out from the darkness toward light again. Job's friends came and sat with him silently for seven days as he suffered. God does not say he will remove all heartache, at least not in this world, but God does promise to be present in our suffering. These promises tear down the walls of isolation often associated with depression and allow the light to creep in and warm us again.

Often, support group leaders will start with a prayer and a reading. Participants share part of their week with each other. Two important questions may be asked: "What has helped you through this week?" and "What are you looking forward to?" Confidentiality is essential. Emphasis is not focused on the depression, but on the healing taking place. All successes, no matter how small, are celebrated.

SEEK THE SPECIAL GIFTS YOUR CHURCH HAS TO OFFER THE DEPRESSED PERSON

We need our churches to be praying communities where gentle listening gives permission to talk about and pray about our hurts. Aside from providing pastoral counseling, your church can provide an environment of acceptance and grace. Ask for holy communion. This simple act unites us with God who pours balm over our battered self-esteem. Loved and cherished, we know God acknowledges our suffering and continues to claim us as God's child in spite of our own perceived brokenness. The simple action of holding out one's hand to receive the bread is an important step toward wholeness. We are acknowledging our need and our faith in our God to meet us even at our weakest points.

MEET WITH YOUR PASTOR

Most pastors are trained to provide care for people in a variety of difficult situations. Prayer both before and after a time together helps both clergy and parishioner remember who guides them. Spiritual guidance or direction can help a person deal with issues of abandonment ("God wasn't there for me . . .") and low self-esteem often associated with depression. It can provide an opportunity for confession and forgiveness for those working through issues of guilt and shame. And in our weakness, when we can't pray for ourselves, the caregivers in our family of faith can give us the assurance that others are praying for us. We are allowed to float in the grace and goodness of God, being assured of Jesus' unrelenting love for us. These prayers are bright lights in darkened times. Later, as healing comes, times of spiritual guidance become less and less about us and our woes and more about God's love. We cultivate some serious listening to the still, small voice of God, not the loud, hurt voice we're so used to. If the hurt is still too great, too loud, perhaps it's still a time to seek out professional counseling and return to spiritual direction later when you are more whole.

MANY FIND COMFORT IN FAMILIAR HYMNS OR SONGS OF WORSHIP

One woman, who experienced a deep depression and now leads a depression support group in her church, shared how the words of a hymn "Jesus, Savior, pilot me over life's tempestuous sea . . ." helped her through her dark moments. Leaning on familiar songs, prayers, or inspiring devotions allows our bodies to rest, our minds to focus, and our spirits to begin to sing again.

These first steps acknowledge our need for others. While depression often seeks to disconnect us from those around us, support groups, and our own community of faith—with its tradition of shared prayer, communion, and fellowship—can provide us with a love that will not let us go. Along with medical care, professional counseling, and spiritual guidance, reaching out to others allows us once again to began to help ourselves, too.

§ Chapter Four §
What More Can I Do to Help Myself?

When a person feels depressed, healthy habits such as physical activity, prayer, and talking to a pastor, counselor, or therapist seem hard to do. It's common to think that one's problems are simply too overwhelming to allow for these things. The depressed person feels too tired, too distracted, too busy, too hopeless. Yet it is at such times that even a modest beginning may count as a very great success!

EXERCISE

The director of a mental health clinic told us that "regular aerobic exercise is worth as much value in dealing with mild depression as the same amount of time spent in psychoanalysis." Walking or running for half an hour at least three times a week over several months, even without other therapeutic help, has been shown to give relief from depression to more than half of those participating in national studies. Besides helping restore a positive chemical balance to the brain, benefits include a more positive self-image, relief from frustrations and anger, and a distraction from one's worries.[3]

When is the next time you could reasonably go for a modest walk, run, jog, or stroll with your wheelchair? How about when you next put this book down? Why not now? This book will be right where you put it when you get back.

All right, so you didn't go right away. But plan a time right now.

If you are already physically active, congratulations. If not, you have some inertia to overcome. Inertia is the tendency for things that are moving to keep moving and things that are stationary to remain stationary, sedentary. And eventually your physical lethargy will give you a brooding body to match the state of your emotions. Exercise. Then celebrate it. And then exercise. Then celebrate. Just starting may be the hardest, smartest, and bravest thing you do today!

$\mathcal{P}$RAY

For some of us, spiritual exercise seems even harder to initiate than physical exercise. The jumbled power of our emotions may seem like a thicket of brambles too tangled for prayer. As a pastor, I (David) am, in a sense, a professional pray-er. But my experiences with depression have brought times when the words didn't come easily. At such times, when our thoughts do no more than bend toward God, I believe our powerful emotions, transmitted by the Spirit, carry the message quite articulately in prayer to a God who always hears and who always cares.

"And the Holy Spirit helps us in our distress. For we don't even know what we should pray for, nor how we should pray. But the Holy Spirit prays for us with groanings that cannot be expressed in words" (Romans 8:26).

The greatest gift of prayer I've ever received came to me during the latter of two significant depression episodes I've experienced in my life, one in the midst of a war and the other right on schedule for midlife crisis (though I prefer to call it midlife *opportunity time*).

I had been a pastor for more than a decade when way too many grieving experiences bunched up on me within just a few months. Even normal activities became difficult. In that particular kind of distress, I literally did not know how to pray, so I had to trust that my inner groanings were getting through. But I also began to pray the Jesus Prayer: "Lord Jesus Christ, Son of God, have mercy on me, a sinner." I dredged up the prayer from years earlier when I had read *The Way of a Pilgrim,* a Russian spiritual classic.

The book and the prayer have been a great blessing for centuries, especially for our sisters and brothers in the Eastern Orthodox Church. At first I prayed it sporadically: "Lord Jesus Christ, Son of God, have mercy on me, a sinner." It had an effect on me similar to hitting a restart button on a computer. It put the essentials—key elements of life's operating system—back into their proper order. Who the Savior is. Who I am in relation to Christ. "Lord Jesus Christ, Son of God, have mercy on me, a sinner."

I found myself turning to this prayer more and more often. Eventually, I allowed myself to pray the Jesus Prayer whenever I heard a bell or horn or alarm. "Lord Jesus Christ, Son of God, have mercy on me, a sinner." I even set my digital watch to chime on the hour so I could pray, "Lord Jesus Christ, Son of God, have mercy on me, a sinner." Every hour on the hour, oh so quietly and privately, I clung to a prayer that allowed me to cling to my Savior. It was the Lord who drew me into this prayer. It didn't require any original thinking on my part. Nothing eloquent. Just a few simple words: "Lord Jesus Christ, Son of God, have mercy on me, a sinner."

Very healing. You'll find yourself treasuring each word. Pray it as you breathe. Inhale "Lord Jesus Christ . . ." as though you physically take in the grace of his presence. Exhale ". . . Son of God . . ." as you remember that God breathed the living Word into this world. Inhale ". . . have mercy on me . . ." taking in the truth that God does not punish us as we deserve. Exhale ". . . a sinner." It's your call whether you have sin to confess or if this is simply an ending sigh of relief. Turn to books of prayers and hymns; luxuriate in their beautiful wisdom.

READ THE WORD OF GOD

One of the common experiences of depression is the circular nature of the dark thoughts. When one feels depressed, the whole world seems darker. This is where one's spiritual life, simple or limited though it may be, becomes critical. Contact with the living God, the comforter Holy Spirit, brings the gift of light into one's thoughts that come from outside of, and are other than, one's own thoughts. We crave something, something to break in on the negative circular pattern where we get depressed about being depressed, so we get further depressed. It doesn't take much of a spark or flame to interrupt true darkness. That's where the light from God's written Word comes in.

During my first depression episode, lasting a number of months while I was in Southeast Asia at the end of the Vietnam War, I (David) was in my early twenties, working for the hyper-secret National Security Agency and almost totally unfamiliar with the Bible. It seemed that many otherwise rational people in that time and place did not have very good mental health. In fact, I would learn much later that hospital psych floors tend to draw many normal people responding quite normally to very abnormal situations at home or elsewhere in their lives. The war was a setting where it was sanity that seemed crazy.

One day, in a dangerous, spiraling, inner darkness, I started reading the Bible. It was literally a race with the clock to find something to live for. My job could not have been more stressful as we gathered front-line intelligence during the fall of South Vietnam. Then I'd race back to my barracks, plop into my papasan chair, and read the Bible, sometimes for hours.

One night a friend, Don, and I sat up all night reading all 150 psalms aloud and discussing most of them. The sheer scope of the inner human drama in the psalms was awesome. And how many laments we found! Griping followed by dark thoughts followed by paranoia followed by more griping followed by . . .

hope in almost every case! Laments can draw hurting people into a relationship with God, helping to construct a forward-looking hope. The Scriptures were retooling my brain.

I remember precisely where I was three weeks later when I halted in the middle of the street near my barracks as I realized with a shock, "I'm not even thinking the same any more!" Something had broken in on my cloudy ruminations. Something was different. And different, in this case, was very good.

Structure can be very helpful and therapeutic when we're depressed. Exercise, prayer, reading God's Word, and other forms of spiritual seeking are especially critical at such times. Small steps—especially first steps in these areas—can be enormously helpful. Further steps are even better. Don't evaluate the success of these activities by how they make you feel. Feelings are sometimes bound and gagged by depression, unable to attest to the merits of any therapy, especially in spiritual things. Simply do what you are able that others have found to work, celebrate the small steps, keep at it, and trust that the good will come.

Lectio Divina

In the sixth century, when few could read and fewer actually owned books, there was a greater sense of emotional involvement in reading/hearing the scriptures. Saint Benedict began a practice that is continued in Benedictine communities and among Christians of many backgrounds to this day: lectio divina [LEK-tsee-oh di-VEE-na]. In lectio, one reads the scriptures (or other books that spiritually deepen the reader) very slowly. Like soil that has endured a long winter and is not yet thoroughly thawed, we need the refreshment of the words to linger and be absorbed rather than run off quickly, leaving less chance for growth. This is not to be confused with other kinds of reading for information or entertainment. We come to the reading gently, regularly, ready to receive a divine, healing touch in the deep places of the heart. Ponder the Word of God in your heart, like Mary in Luke 2:19. Then, like Mary, give the word access as she did: "Let it be done to me according to your word" (Luke 1:38b). Lectio is like reading a love letter or poetry where each word is savored, where feelings, memories, and imaginations flare with rich response.

A simple guideline for lectio:

1. Come into the Lord's presence quietly, with humility, ready to receive a word from God. Pray for the Spirit to bless and guide you.

2. Read/hear a few verses of God's Word for ten minutes or so. At times, a single verse will do. If a single word or phrase captures your heart and mind, rest there. Meditate on the Word. Take it in deeply.

3. Finally, select a word or phrase to take with you through the day. Let it come to mind and touch your life often as the day unfolds. Close with thanks for God's presence.

Try lectio divina. You'll see yourself differently. You'll see the world differently.

PRAYER WITH SCRIPTURES

There are passages in the bible that seem written just for this time of depression. Seek them out. Read them using lectio divina, described earlier. Talk about them with others. Jot down a few to carry with you or attach them to the bathroom mirror or a kitchen appliance. Memorize the most meaningful among them and let your mind dwell on them at times when you're prone to mulling over dark thoughts. Consider keeping a spiritual journal during this time of healing.[4] *And especially, read the scriptures as a prelude to prayer.* Probing the depths of depression is a daunting task, but as the Psalmist wrote, "I will incline my ear to a proverb; I will solve my riddle to the music of the harp" (Psalm 49:4).

Naming the Hurts

• Psalm 130—"Out of the depths . . ." De Profundis in Latin. Very profoundly true.

• Psalm 88—An edgy lament, but it keeps the conversation with God going.

• Psalm 38—When you're under the weight of sin (Then see I John 1:8-9).

• Psalm 40:11-13—When you feel hemmed in.

• Psalm 56—When you've been hurt by others (See also Psalms 17 and 35).

• Psalm 4—When you are in distress, anger, or poverty.

• Psalm 55—When you fear death.

• Psalm 22—Even Jesus used this lament. (Note how the mood changes at verse 22.)

• I Corinthians 10:13—God "will not let you be tested beyond your strength . . ." A promise of help with a way out.

• Matthew 7:24-28—Build your life on the Word of God.

The Lord Is Near

• Psalm 30—From mourning and cries to dancing and praise.

• Psalm 73:21-26—Anger toward God makes us bitter, but God is still there.

• Psalm 34:18-19—"The Lord is near to the brokenhearted and saves the crushed in spirit. Many are the afflictions of the righteous, but the Lord rescues them from them all."

• Psalm 85:6-13—"Wilt thou not revive us again?"

• Isaiah 53:4-12, 61:1-3—Meet our Lord Jesus even in the Old Testament.

• I Thessalonians 5:11-22—". . . give thanks in all circumstances . . ."

Words of Hope

• Psalm 27—Waiting is sometimes necessary.

• Psalms 32 and 51—The great Psalms of confession and forgiveness.

• Psalm 42—Has there ever been a more exquisite expression of longing?

• Psalm 28:6-9—The Lord hears our prayers.

• Psalm 71:14-24—Laments almost always end in hope; this one soars!

• Romans 8:26-27—For when you have trouble praying.

• Romans 8:28—This follows the previous verses but deserves to be read on its own.

• James 5:13-15—"Is any one among you suffering?"

• 2 Corinthians 1:2-4, 12:9-10—"My grace is sufficient for you for my power is made perfect in weakness."

• Jeremiah 31:31-34—"I will forgive their iniquity, and remember their sin no more."

• Philippians 4:4-13—Wow. Simply wow.

• Romans 12:15—A word for loved ones of someone who is depressed.

• Matthew 11:28-30—You'll want to memorize this one!

Blessings

• 1 Thessalonians 5:23-24—"May the God of peace himself sanctify you entirely; and may your spirit and soul and body be kept sound and blameless at the coming of our Lord Jesus Christ. The one who calls you is faithful, and he will do this."

• Romans 15:13—"May the God of hope fill you with all joy and peace in believing, so that you may abound in hope by the power of the Holy Spirit."

• 2 Thessalonians 3:16—"Now may the Lord of peace himself give you peace at all times in all ways. The Lord be with all of you."

As you continue in this process of healing:

1. *Be patient.* This is a process that will take some time. Feeling like a failure comes from expecting too much too soon.

2. *Be healthy.* Avoid alcohol and recreational drugs. Temporary highs can lead to persistent lows.

3. *Be active.* Exercise, be social, be involved. Read the Bible and other good books, listen to songs and hymns of faith, keep a spiritual journal, attend worship regularly.

4. *Be prudent.* Know your better times of the day. Set reachable goals. Don't take the world on your shoulders.

Spiritually, in God's grace, the good always comes. No matter how desperate things get in this world, God *always* has the last word. Believe it.

§Chapter Five §
Depression—A Family Perspective

"Rejoice with those who rejoice, weep with those who weep" (Romans 12:15).

"What can I do?" is a common response from loved ones of a person going through depression. In general terms, a family can help a loved one find help and stick to a program of treatment, offer understanding and emotional support, and be good listeners during the journey toward health. The specifics of the help a family can offer depend on the type of depression, the time commitment a person is willing to put into it, and ultimately the level of intimacy one has established with the person with depression. Everybody's story spins out differently.

One thing we do know: depression is a lonely business. "Depression," according to author Parker Palmer when talking about his own experience with the disease, "is the ultimate state of disconnection . . . it deprives one of the relatedness that is the lifeline of every living being." He goes on to explain that depression in not only the ultimate state of disconnection between people, but of feelings and thought, self-image, and the public person we all dress up in the morning and march out the door.

How can a person help someone whose very condition seeks to disconnect them from others? Palmer, in his book *Listen to Your Life,* spoke of friends who meant well but whose very presence during his depression drove him deeper into despair.

For most, depression is a mystery. There are no easy answers, pat solutions, or quick fixes to the problem. What family and friends can offer is a ministry of presence. Presence is the very gift God offers all of us in our suffering. Not to remove us from our suffering, but walk with us through it, reminding us always that *nothing* "will be able to separate us from the love of God in Christ Jesus our Lord" (Romans 8:39b).

A young boy tried to describe to his mother his early signs of depression.

"It's like you're under water, and it's pressing down on you," he said. "It's uncomfortable, the weight of it all. But it's easier to stay there than to try and push back up toward the light."

"When the dark thoughts come," the mother asked naively, "can't you just think of something else? You know . . . not participate."

The boy gave her a sad look. "It's not that easy," he said.

There are no easy answers when it comes to depression. Friends and family are left feeling hopeless and a little afraid. What to do? What to do?

Two parents were grieving. Their son had just committed suicide and their pain ran deep.

"If only he had told us," they lamented. "He didn't even leave a note. How could we know?"

How often we heard similar words when speaking to those whose families had been touched by depression. "If only they could tell us what's wrong. Maybe then we could help."

It would be easier if the depressed person could point and say, "It hurts here." Or, "Rub there, please." But this is a different kind of pain. The fact that there was no note for these sad parents was indeed a note. Depression, at it's worst, robs the person of their ability to tell, to explain or express.

If a depressed person could find the words to describe this strange and foreign land in which they find themselves, what would they say to us? What advice could they offer to the question, "What can I do to help?" Pieced together from those who have been there and returned, they might say something like this:

Don't tell me you know how it feels.
If you've been depressed, you'd know how painful that statement is to me. Unless you've been there, you couldn't possibly know what I'm feeling. Your attempt to identify with me only makes me feel more alone. Even though you mean well, it is better that you are honest with me, acknowledge that you feel powerless and useless to help. Now you will know a little of what I, too, am experiencing.

Don't remind me of what a good person I am.
The depression has denied me the ability to see much good in myself. My self-image has taken a nose dive.

Reminding me of who I used to be only serves to show me how far I've fallen. Accept me for who I am now and love me just the same. Assure me that my depression hasn't changed how you feel about me.

Don't tell me to cheer up.
I can't just cheer up. When you pressure me to act happier, I only feel worse. Pointing out reasons why I should feel happy only adds guilt to the whole mess. It is better that you open my shade to let the sun in and sit with me in its warmth in silence. Telling me "This will make you feel better," will most assuredly predict that I will feel worse.

Please do not offer easy advice.
When you offer advice to me, it is your way of distancing yourself from me. At least you tried, right? If I don't get better, it will be my own fault, not yours. I understand how uncomfortable it is to see me like this. It's okay if you don't know how to fix it. What I really need from you is your presence. Feel powerless with me. Come and be with me in my darkness.

Help me get the help I need.
I really am sick. I need a doctor. I may need to be in a hospital. Help me find the appropriate medical, spiritual, and therapeutic resources for diagnosis and treatment. It may take medicine to help bring back the brain chemicals needed to begin the journey through this. You may need to oversee my medication and general health/hygiene. Depression makes me

forget things like that, or I may not have the strength to do it myself. I may forget to thank you. I'm sorry.

Help our kids express their own feelings.
I know they're confused. Tell them I still love them, even though I may not be able to communicate love as well as I have. It's okay if they are mad at me for changing their lives like this. Help them to know I haven't left them. I'm still here. I'll be well soon.

Learn what you can about depression.
Help me to know that my behaviors are normal for a person with depression. Read about other people's stories. Learn to recognize depressive behavior and thinking. Point them out to me. Then I'll know that you can still see the real me behind the depression.

Reassure me when I make efforts to connect.
It's hard for me to feel like doing anything so when I do it helps me to hear you acknowledge my attempts. Find an encouraging Bible verse, write it down and put it where I can see it. Remind me that God is holding me in the palm of his hand.

Pray for me
Pray with me if I'm open to it. I may not be able to pray myself at this time, but it's comforting to hear your voice raised on my behalf. Read to me from the Bible or other helpful resources. The Psalms are full of laments. They will help me not feel so alone in my suffering.

Try not to take my depression personally.
Neither one of us caused this to happen. I know you sometimes feel guilty for not doing or saying something sooner. We did the best we could with the knowledge we had. I know you're picking up a lot of loose pieces for me now. Never forget how important you are to me. Thank you for staying with me during this dark time. Your love gives me courage and strength to keep trying.

Don't try to go it alone.
Just as I need your presence in my life, you need God's presence in yours. Especially now. Ask friends to pray for us. Find a counselor or support group from which to draw encouragement. I need you to be strong. This is a difficult time for all of us. Look for support.

A ministry of presence shared with a depressed person gives non-judgmental support and a strong shoulder to make the burden light. The gift of presence is most often shared in silence, with no expectations or response required. Parker Palmer spoke of a friend who came once a week, knelt before him to remove his shoes and rubbed his feet. His friend had found the only spot on Palmer's body where he still could feel. A gift of grace reminiscent of the last supper. Servanthood at its best.

Many a former depressed person shared little things a spouse or friend had done during their illness that were beneficial to them. One woman said the thing that helped her the most during her depression was her husband's cheerful whistling in the morning. Another liked to listen to the voice of his friend while he read the Psalms.

A young girl, having trouble sleeping at night because of her dark thoughts, got to have the dog in her bed. It helped. Skipper supplied an unending source of unconditional love as well as a few degrees of body heat, a connection to another living thing during late night hours. Other small and helpful actions: fresh flowers, clean sheets, soothing music on the radio. All placed into the environment without comments or expectation. Gifts of grace helping to reestablish a connection. Fragile threads between darkness and light.

It is important in dealing with the depressed person that those with whom they live are not forgotten. If you are the support person for someone going through a depression, it is important that you are gentle with yourself. Give yourself the needed time to recuperate both physically and mentally each day. Accept kindnesses when they are offered. They will strengthen you, and you will soon be able to offer them back.

It is also important not to deny what is happening or deny your own feelings of frustration and fear. Denial stops us from acknowledging our need for help. Denying depression or any emotion, in ourselves and others, never helps; it only hurts. Be open enough to recognize what is happening and not push it away. Acknowledging brokenness in any form is the first step toward healing for all involved.

OTHER RESOURCES FROM AUGSBURG

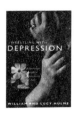

Wrestling with Depression
by William and Lucy Hulme
128 pages, ISBN 0-8066-2699-2

To the twenty million Americans who
suffer from depression, the authors bring
the promise of hope and healing.

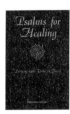

Psalms for Healing by Gretchen Person
170 pages, ISBN 0-8066-4161-4

A thoughtful collection of psalms and
prayers for those who seek healing.

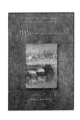

When You Lose Your Job
by Donna Bennett
48 pages, ISBN 0-8066-4362-5

The transition from work to joblessness
and back to work is a stressful one.
Donna Bennett offers a wealth of advice
in making that transition smoothly.

Available wherever books are sold.
To order these books directly, contact:
1-800-328-4648 • www.augsburgfortress.org
Augsburg Fortress, Publishers
P.O. Box 1209, Minneapolis, MN 55440-1209